Juicing for Beginners

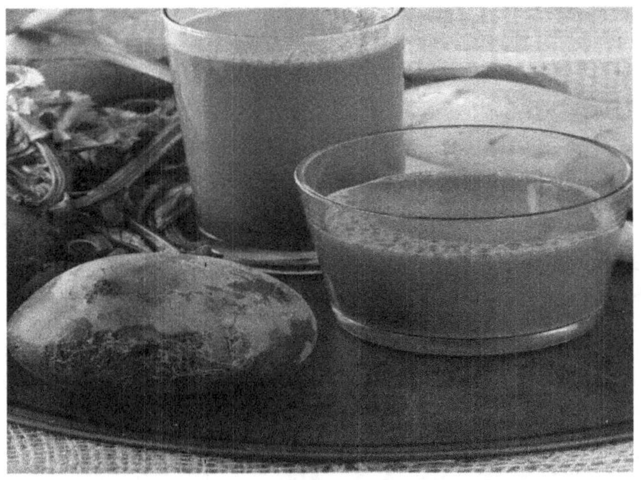

The Essential Guide to Natural Juices
Recipes for Effective Weight Loss
and Well-Being

Isaac Hendricks

Table of Contents

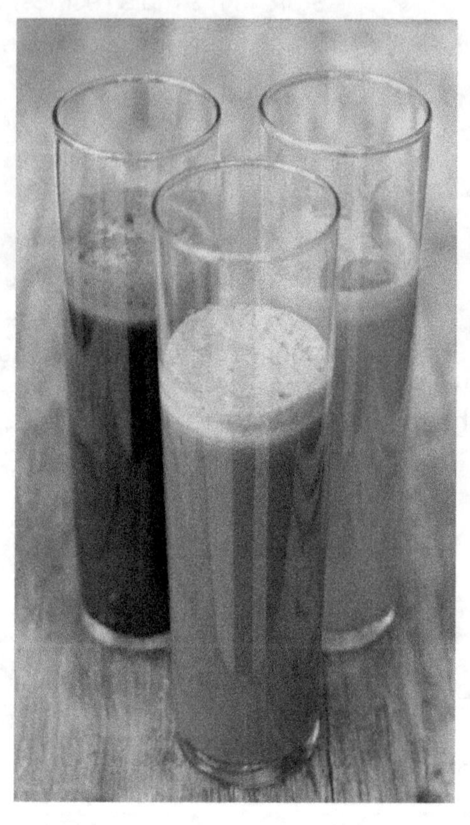

8

INTRODUCTION

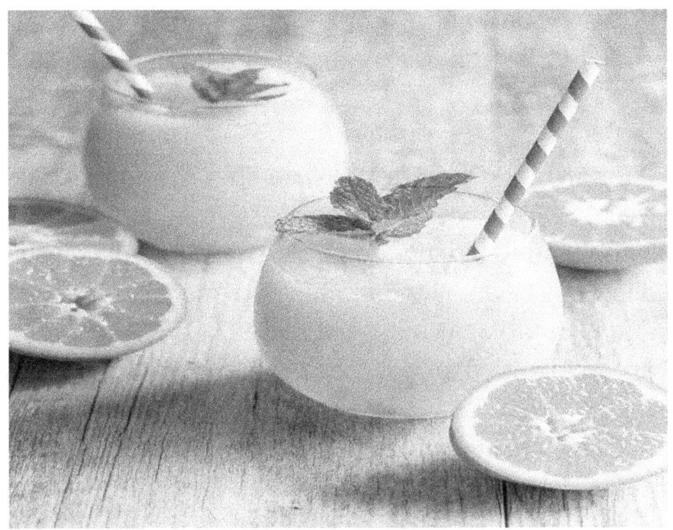

Brief Overview of Juicing and its Benefits

Juicing is the process of extracting the liquid content, or juice, from fruits and vegetables using a specialised machine called a juicer. This process separates the pulp and fibre from the juice, resulting in a concentrated source of vitamins, minerals, and other nutrients.

Juicing has grown in popularity in recent years because to the multiple health benefits it provides. Here are some of the most significant advantages of incorporating juicing into your diet:

1. Increased Nutrient Absorption: When we eat whole fruits and vegetables, our bodies have to work hard to break down the fibre and extract the nutrients. Juicing removes the fibre, making it easier for our bodies to absorb the nutrients quickly and efficiently.

2. Improved Digestion: While fibre is essential for maintaining a healthy digestive system, too much of it can lead to bloating, gas, and discomfort. Juicing allows us to enjoy the nutritional benefits of fruits and vegetables without the added fiber, making it an excellent option for those with digestive issues.

3. Boosts Energy Levels: Juices are packed with natural sugars that provide a quick burst of energy. This makes them an excellent pre-workout or midday pick-me-up.

4. Promotes Weight Loss: Juices are low in calories and high in nutrients, making them an excellent option for those looking to lose weight. They can also help curb cravings and reduce overall calorie intake.

5. Enhances Skin Health: Many fruits and vegetables contain antioxidants that help protect our skin from damage caused by free radicals. Juicing allows us to consume large amounts of these antioxidants in a single serving, promoting healthy, radiant skin.

6. Reduces Inflammation: Many common health issues, such as arthritis and asthma, are caused by inflammation in the body. Juicing can help reduce inflammation by providing anti-inflammatory nutrients such as ginger, turmeric, and leafy greens.

7. Promotes Hydration: Many fruits and vegetables contain high water content, making them an excellent way to stay hydrated throughout the day. Juices can also help replenish electrolytes lost during exercise or illness.

In conclusion, juicing offers numerous health benefits that make it an excellent addition to any diet. Whether you're looking to boost your energy levels, improve your digestion, or promote overall health and wellness, incorporating juicing into your routine is an excellent choice!

Who should try juicing?

Juicing has grown in popularity in recent years as a result of its multiple health benefits. While it's true that anyone can enjoy the benefits of juicing, there are certain individuals who may find it particularly beneficial. Here are a few people who should consider trying juicing:

- Those with busy lifestyles: In today's fast-paced world, it can be challenging to find the time to prepare healthy meals.

Juicing offers a quick and easy way to consume a large amount of nutrients in a short amount of time. By drinking a glass of fresh juice, you can provide your body with the essential vitamins and minerals it needs to function optimally.

- People with digestive issues: Juicing can be an excellent way to soothe digestive issues such as bloating, constipation, and indigestion. By consuming fresh fruits and vegetables in their raw form, you can provide your body with the fibre it needs to promote healthy digestion. Additionally, certain fruits and vegetables such as ginger, lemon, and cucumber have natural anti-inflammatory properties that can help soothe digestive discomfort.

- Athletes and fitness enthusiasts: Juicing can be an excellent way for athletes and fitness enthusiasts to replenish their bodies after a workout. Fresh fruit and vegetable juices are packed with electrolytes, which can help replenish fluids lost during exercise. Additionally, certain fruits and vegetables such as beets and spinach are rich in nitrates, which can help improve athletic performance by increasing blood flow and oxygen delivery to the muscles.

- Individuals looking to lose weight: Juicing can be an effective way to lose weight by providing your body with the nutrients it needs without the excess calories found in solid foods. By consuming fresh fruit and vegetable juices, you can provide your body with the vitamins and minerals it needs while also reducing your overall calorie intake. Additionally, certain fruits and vegetables such as celery and cucumber are low in calories but high in fibre, making them an excellent choice for those looking to lose weight.

- People with chronic health conditions: Juicing can be an effective way for individuals with chronic health conditions such as diabetes, high blood pressure, or heart disease to manage their symptoms. By consuming fresh fruit and vegetable juices, you can provide your body with the nutrients it needs while also reducing your overall intake of sugar, salt, and unhealthy fats found in processed foods. Additionally, certain fruits and vegetables such as berries and leafy greens are rich in antioxidants, which can help reduce inflammation and improve overall health.

In conclusion, while anyone can enjoy the benefits of juicing, there are certain individuals who may find it particularly beneficial. Whether you're looking to improve your digestion, boost your athletic performance, or manage a chronic health condition, juicing offers a quick and easy way to provide your body with the nutrients it needs to function optimally. So why not give it a try? Your body will thank you!

How to use this guide

This guide is designed to help beginners navigate the world of juicing, providing tips and tricks to help you get started and make the most of your new juicer. Here's how to use this guide:

1. Read the Introduction: The introduction provides an overview of what juicing is, its benefits, and why you might want to start juicing. It's a great place to start if you're new to juicing and want to learn more about what it's all about.

2. Choose Your Juicer: The next section of the guide helps you choose the right juicer for your needs. Whether you're on a budget or looking for a high-end model, there's a juicer out there that's right for you. This section will help you narrow down your options and make an informed decision.

3. Preparing Your Produce: Before you start juicing, it's important to prepare your produce properly. This section covers everything from washing and chopping your fruits and vegetables to storing them properly. Follow these tips to ensure that your produce is fresh, clean, and ready to be juiced.

4. Basic Juice Recipes: If you're not sure where to start when it comes to creating your own juice recipes, this section is for you. It includes a variety of simple, delicious juice recipes that are perfect for beginners. Test them out and see which ones you prefer!

5. Advanced Juice Recipes: Once you've mastered the basics, it's time to get creative with your juice recipes. This section includes more advanced recipes that incorporate a variety of fruits and vegetables, as well as some unexpected ingredients like ginger and turmeric. Don't be afraid to try new things and explore!

6. Troubleshooting Common Issues: Juicing can be a bit tricky at first, especially if you're new to it. This section covers some common issues that beginners may encounter, such as clogging or foaming, and provides tips on how to fix them. Don't let these problems discourage you – with a little troubleshooting, you can overcome them and enjoy delicious, healthy juice every time!

7. Tips for Maximising Nutrition: Juicing is a great way to get a lot of nutrients into your body quickly and easily. This section provides tips on how to maximise the nutrition content of your juice, such as using organic produce and adding superfoods like chia seeds or spirulina. By following these tips, you can ensure that your juice is not only delicious but also packed with nutrients!

8. How Often Should You Juice?: Finally, this section covers how often you should be juicing in order to reap the full benefits of this healthy habit. Whether you're just starting out or have been juicing for a while, this information will help you create a juicing routine that works for you!

CHAPTER ONE

Getting Started with Juicing

Choosing the Right Juicer for Your Needs

When it comes to choosing the right juicer for your needs, there are several factors to consider. Here are some key points to help you make an informed decision:

Type of Juicer:

There are three main types of juicers: centrifugal, masticating, and cold-press. Centrifugal juicers are fast and efficient, but they generate more heat and oxidation, which can affect the nutritional value of the juice. Masticating juicers, also known as slow juicers, operate at a lower speed and produce less heat, resulting in a higher nutrient content and longer shelf life. Cold-press juicers use hydraulic pressure to extract juice without generating heat or oxidation, resulting in the highest nutrient content and longest shelf life.

Juicing Needs:

Consider what types of produce you plan to juice most frequently. If you prefer softer fruits and vegetables like berries, grapes, and leafy greens, a masticating juicer may be a better choice as it can handle these items more easily. If you prefer harder fruits and vegetables like apples, carrots, and beets, a centrifugal juicer may be more suitable as it can handle these items more efficiently.

Budget:

Juicers can range from a few hundred dollars to several thousand dollars. Consider your budget and prioritise features that are most important to you. For example, if you're on a tight budget, a basic centrifugal juicer may be sufficient for your needs. If you're willing to spend more, a high-end cold-press juicer may offer additional features and benefits.

Ease of Use:

Consider how easy the juicer is to clean and operate. Some models have dishwasher-safe parts for easy cleanup, while others require more manual cleaning. Some models also have intuitive controls and user-friendly interfaces for easy operation.

Warranty:

Look for a juicer with a strong warranty to protect your investment. A longer warranty typically indicates higher quality and durability.

Brand Reputation:

Research the reputation of the brand before making your purchase. Look for brands with a proven track record of producing high-quality juicers that stand the test of time.

By considering these factors, you can choose the right juicer for your needs and enjoy fresh, nutrient-rich juice at home!

Preparing your fruits and vegetables

Juicing is a popular way to consume fruits and vegetables in their most nutrient-dense form. It allows you to pack a lot of vitamins, minerals, and enzymes into a single glass, making it an excellent choice for those looking to improve their health and wellbeing. However, preparing your fruits and vegetables for juicing can be a bit daunting, especially for beginners. Here are some pointers to get you started:

1. <u>Wash your produce thoroughly:</u> Before you start juicing, make sure to wash your fruits and vegetables thoroughly with water. This will get rid of any dirt, pesticides, or microorganisms that might be on the surface.

2. <u>Remove any inedible parts:</u> Cut off any stems, leaves, or cores that are not edible. This will ensure that your juice is smooth and easy to drink.

3. <u>Cut your produce into small pieces:</u> To make the juicing process easier and more efficient, cut your

fruits and vegetables into small pieces that will fit into the juicer's chute. This will also help to prevent clogging and ensure that all the juice is extracted.

4. Alternate hard and soft produce: To prevent your juicer from getting clogged, alternate between hard and soft produce. For example, start with a few carrots, followed by an apple or a cucumber. This will help to keep the machine running smoothly and prevent any jams or blockages.

5. Experiment with different combinations: Don't be afraid to try out different combinations of fruits and vegetables to find what you like best. Some popular combinations include carrot-orange, spinach-kale-apple, and beet-carrot-ginger. You can also add some lemon or lime juice for a tangy flavour or a pinch of cayenne pepper for a spicy kick.

6. Store your juice properly: Once you've made your juice, store it in an airtight container in the refrigerator for up to 24 hours. Make sure to give it a good shake before drinking as the sediment may settle at the bottom over time.

7. Clean your juicer thoroughly: After each use, disassemble your juicer and clean all the parts thoroughly with water and soap. This will help to prevent any bacteria from growing inside the machine and ensure that it lasts for many years to come.

By following these tips, you'll be able to prepare your fruits and vegetables for juicing like a pro! Happy juicing!

Tips for cleaning and maintaining your juicer

Juicers are a great addition to any healthy lifestyle, but they require proper cleaning and maintenance to ensure they continue to function efficiently and hygienically. Here are some tips for cleaning and maintaining your juicer:

- Clean your juicer immediately after use: This will prevent any leftover pulp or juice from drying and becoming difficult to remove. Rinse all parts with warm water and use a soft-bristled brush to remove any remaining pulp.

- Disassemble your juicer for cleaning: Most juicers can be easily disassembled for thorough cleaning. This will allow you to reach all the nooks and crannies where pulp and juice can accumulate.

- Use a citrus-based cleaner: Citrus-based cleaners like lemon or lime juice can help remove any stubborn stains or residue from your juicer. Simply squeeze half a lemon or lime into the juicer and run it through the machine.

- Clean the filter screen: The filter screen is an important part of your juicer that prevents pulp from passing through into the juice. It can become clogged with pulp over time, so it's essential to clean it regularly. Use a soft-bristled brush to gently scrub the screen, or remove it and wash it in warm soapy water.

- Store your juicer properly: After cleaning, make sure to dry all parts thoroughly before storing them away. This will prevent any mould or bacteria from growing in damp areas. Store your juicer in a cool, dry place away from direct sunlight.

- Regularly inspect the blades: Over time, the blades on your juicer may become dull or damaged, which can affect the quality of your juice. Inspect the blades regularly and replace them if necessary.

- Lubricate moving parts: Some juicers have moving parts that require lubrication to ensure they continue to function smoothly. Check your user manual for specific instructions on how often and how to lubricate these parts.

By following these tips, you can ensure that your juicer continues to function efficiently and hygienically for years to come!

Troubleshooting common issues

Juicing is a popular trend in the health and wellness industry, as it allows individuals to consume large amounts of nutrients and vitamins in a concentrated form. However, for beginners, the process of juicing can be daunting, as it involves using complex machinery and understanding the intricacies of the ingredients. In this article, we will discuss some common issues that beginners may encounter while juicing and provide solutions to help them overcome these challenges.

Juicer not producing enough juice

One of the most common issues that beginners face is not getting enough juice from their fruits and vegetables. This can be due to a few reasons, such as using old or wilted produce, not washing the produce properly, or not cutting it into small enough pieces.

To overcome this issue, make sure to use fresh and crisp produce that is free from any mould or spoilage. To remove any dirt or bacteria, thoroughly wash the vegetables under running water. Cut the produce into small pieces, especially for leafy greens like spinach and kale, as they can clog the juicer if they are too large.

Juice is too thick or too thin

Another issue that beginners may encounter is that their juice is either too thick or too thin. This can be due to using too much or too little water in the juicer, respectively.

To make the juice thicker, use less water in the juicer. Begin with a tiny amount of water and gradually add more until the appropriate consistency is reached. To make the juice thinner, use more water in the juicer. This will help to dilute the juice and make it easier to drink.

Juice has an unpleasant taste or odour

Some beginners may find that their juice has an unpleasant taste or odour, which can be due to using produce that is past its prime or not storing it properly. This can also be due to using too much of a particular ingredient, such as ginger or garlic, which can overpower the other flavours in the juice.

To overcome this issue, use fresh produce that is free from any spoilage or mould. Store your produce properly in the refrigerator to prevent it from going bad prematurely. Use a variety of ingredients in your juice to balance out the flavours and prevent any one ingredient from dominating the taste.

Some beginners may find that their juice contains pulp or sediment, which can be due to using a slow juicer or not straining the juice properly. This can also be due to using too many seeds or fibrous materials in the juice, such as celery or cucumber seeds.

To overcome this issue, use a high-speed juicer or a centrifugal juicer to extract more juice and less pulp from your fruits and vegetables. Strain the juice through a fine mesh sieve or cheesecloth to remove any remaining pulp or sediment. Remove any seeds or fibrous materials from your fruits and vegetables before juicing them to prevent them from getting caught in the juicer and causing clogs.

Some beginners may find that their juice is not nutritious enough, as they are not including enough fruits and vegetables with high nutrient content in their recipes. This can also be due to using too many low-nutrient fruits like apples and pears in their recipes.

To overcome this issue, focus on including more leafy greens like spinach and kale in your recipes, as they are packed with vitamins and minerals. Use a variety of fruits and vegetables with high nutrient content like carrots, beets, ginger, and turmeric to create a well-rounded and nutritious juice recipe.

Limit your intake of low-nutrient fruits like apples and pears to prevent them from overpowering the other flavours in your recipe.

CHAPTER TWO

Basic Juice Recipes for Beginners

Green Juice (spinach, cucumber, apple, lemon)

Green juice is a refreshing and healthy beverage that is packed with essential vitamins, minerals, and antioxidants. It's a great way to start your day, as it provides your body with the nutrients it needs to function optimally. In this article, we'll be discussing a basic green juice recipe that is perfect for beginners.

Ingredients:
- 1 cup spinach
- 1 medium-sized cucumber
- 1 medium-sized apple
- 1 lemon (juiced)

Instructions:
1. Thoroughly wash all of the ingredients under running water.
2. Cut the cucumber into small pieces and remove the seeds.
3. Cut the apple into quarters and remove the core.
4. Add the spinach, cucumber, and apple to a juicer.
5. Squeeze the lemon juice into the juicer.

6. Turn on the juicer and let it run until all the ingredients have been juiced.
7. Pour the green juice into a glass and serve immediately.

Spinach: Spinach is an excellent source of iron, calcium, and vitamins A, C, and K. It's also low in calories and high in fibre, making it a great addition to any green juice recipe.

Cucumber: Cucumbers are rich in water content, which makes them an excellent hydrating ingredient for green juice. They're also high in vitamins C and K and low in calories.

Apple: Apples add a touch of sweetness to green juice, making it more palatable for beginners who may find green juice too bitter at first. They're also rich in fibre, vitamins C and K, and antioxidants like flavonoids and polyphenols.

Lemon: Lemons add a tangy flavour to green juice and also provide a good source of vitamin C, which helps boost your immune system. They're also rich in antioxidants like flavonoids and limonoids that have anti-inflammatory properties.

Benefits of Green Juice:

1. Boosts energy levels: Green juice provides your body with a quick burst of energy due to its high nutrient content. It's an excellent alternative to sugary drinks or coffee that can give you a quick energy boost but also lead to crashes later on.

2. *Promotes weight loss:* Green juice is low in calories but high in fibre, which helps keep you feeling full for longer periods of time. This can help you avoid overeating and promote weight loss over time.

3. *Improves digestion:* The fibre content in green juice helps promote healthy digestion by keeping your bowels regular and preventing constipation. It also helps prevent bloating and gas due to its low sugar content.

4. *Boosts immunity:* Green juice is rich in vitamins C and K, which are essential for maintaining a healthy immune system. These vitamins help protect your body from infection and disease by promoting the production of white blood cells that fight off pathogens.

5. *Promotes healthy skin:* Green juice is rich in antioxidants like vitamin C, flavonoids, and polyphenols that help protect your skin from damage caused by free radicals. These antioxidants also help promote healthy collagen production, which leads to firmer, more youthful-looking skin over time.

Carrot and ginger juice (carrots, ginger, lemon)

Carrot and ginger juice, made with fresh carrots, ginger, and lemon, is a delicious and healthy drink that's perfect for beginners who are new to juicing. This simple recipe is packed with nutrients and offers a range of health benefits.

Carrots are rich in beta-carotene, a compound that the body converts into vitamin A. This vitamin is essential for maintaining healthy eyesight, skin, and bones. Carrots also contain fibre, potassium, and vitamin C.

Ginger is known for its anti-inflammatory properties and can help to soothe an upset stomach. It also has a warming effect on the body, making it a great choice for colder months.

Lemon adds a tart and refreshing flavour to the juice, as well as vitamin C and antioxidants.

To make carrot and ginger juice, you'll need:

- 4 medium-sized carrots, washed and peeled
- 1 inch piece peeled and chopped fresh ginger
- 1 lemon, peeled and seeded

Here's how to make it:

1. Wash all of your ingredients thoroughly to remove any dirt or debris. Peel the carrots and ginger using a vegetable peeler or knife. Remove the seeds from the lemon and cut it in half.

2. Cut the carrots into small pieces that will fit into your juicer's chute. Chop the ginger into smaller pieces as well to ensure that it juices easily.

3. Place the carrots, ginger, and lemon into your juicer in the order listed. If you have a slow juicer, you may want to juice the carrots first to extract as much juice as possible before adding the other ingredients.

4. Turn on your juicer and let it run until all of the ingredients have been fully juiced. You may need to stop the machine occasionally to push down any remaining pulp or fibres.

5. Pour the juice into a glass or pitcher and serve immediately. You can add ice cubes or water to dilute the juice if you prefer a less concentrated drink.

Carrot and ginger juice is a delicious and healthy choice for beginners who are new to juicing. It's packed with nutrients and offers a range of health benefits that will leave you feeling refreshed and energised. Give it a try today!

Orange and beet juice (oranges, beets, lemon)

Orange and Beet Juice: A Delightful and Nutritious Basic Juice Recipe for Beginners

Juicing is a healthy and delicious way to incorporate more fruits and vegetables into your diet. If you're new to juicing, it's best to start with simple recipes that are easy to prepare and packed with essential nutrients. In this article, we'll share a basic juice recipe that combines the sweetness of oranges with the earthy flavour of beets, all blended with a touch of lemon for a refreshing and nutritious drink.

Ingredients:
- 4 medium-sized oranges, peeled
- 2 medium-sized beets, peeled and chopped
- 1 lemon, peeled

Instructions:
1. Wash all the fruits and vegetables thoroughly.
2. Peel the oranges and chop them into small pieces.
3. Peel the beets and chop them into small pieces as well.
4. Cut the lemon in half and remove any seeds.
5. Add all the ingredients into a juicer, starting with the oranges, followed by the beets, and finally the lemon.

6. Turn on the juicer and let it run until all the ingredients are fully extracted.

7. Pour the juice into a glass and serve immediately.

8. Enjoy your delicious and nutritious orange and beet juice!

Benefits of Orange and Beet Juice:

Oranges are rich in vitamin C, which helps boost the immune system, while beets are packed with antioxidants, fibre, and potassium that promote heart health and aid in digestion. Lemon adds a tangy flavour to the juice while also providing vitamin C and alkalizing properties that help balance the body's pH level. Together, these ingredients make for a refreshing and nutrient-dense drink that's perfect for starting your day or as a healthy snack anytime of the day!

Pineapple and kale juice (pineapple, kale, lemon)

Pineapple and kale juice is a refreshing and healthy drink that is perfect for beginners who are new to the world of juicing. This basic recipe combines the sweetness of pineapple with the nutrient-rich goodness of kale and a squeeze of lemon, creating a delicious and nourishing beverage that is packed with vitamins and minerals.

Ingredients:

- 1 medium-sized pineapple, peeled and chopped

- 2 cups of kale leaves, washed and chopped
- 1 lemon, juiced

Instructions:
1. Wash all ingredients thoroughly to remove any dirt or debris.
2. Peel the pineapple and chop it into small pieces that will fit easily into your juicer.
3. Wash the kale leaves thoroughly and remove the tough stems. Chop the leaves into small pieces.
4. Squeeze the lemon to extract its juice.
5. Add the pineapple, kale, and lemon juice to your juicer in the order listed.
6. Turn on your juicer and let it run until all the ingredients have been processed.
7. Pour the juice into a glass and serve immediately.

Benefits of Pineapple and Kale Juice:

Pineapple contains a high concentration of vitamin C, which helps to improve the immune system and maintain healthy skin. Bromelain, an enzyme that assists digestion and lowers inflammation, is also present. Kale is a superfood that is packed with vitamins A, C, and K, as well as iron and calcium. Lemon adds a tangy flavour to the juice while also providing vitamin C and antioxidants. Together, these ingredients make for a delicious and nutritious drink that is perfect for anyone looking to start their juicing journey on a healthy note!

Watermelon and mint juice (watermelon, mint leaves)

Watermelon and mint juice is a refreshing and healthy beverage that's perfect for hot summer days. This simple recipe is easy to make and requires only two ingredients: watermelon and fresh mint leaves. Here's how to make it:

Ingredients:
- 4 cups of seedless watermelon, cubed
- 1/4 cup of fresh mint leaves
- Ice (optional)

Instructions:
1. Wash the watermelon and mint leaves thoroughly.
2. Cut the watermelon into small cubes and remove the seeds if necessary.
3. Add the watermelon cubes and mint leaves to a blender.
4. Blend until the mixture is smooth and creamy.
5. Pour the juice into a glass filled with ice (optional).
6. Garnish with additional mint leaves and serve immediately.

This basic juice recipe is perfect for beginners because it requires only two ingredients and is easy to prepare. Watermelon is rich in vitamins A and C, as well as potassium, while mint leaves are known for their soothing and refreshing properties.

Together, they create a delicious and healthy drink that's perfect for quenching your thirst on a hot day. Enjoy!

CHAPTER THREE

How to Store and Preserve Your Juices

Storing freshly made juice in the fridge

Storing freshly made juice in the fridge is a great way to preserve its nutrients and flavour for longer periods. However, it's essential to follow some simple guidelines to ensure that your juice stays fresh and safe to drink.

Here are some tips for storing freshly made juice in the fridge:

Use clean containers

Always use clean and sterile containers to store your juice. Wash the containers thoroughly with soap and hot water before filling them with juice. This will prevent any bacteria from growing in the container and spoiling the juice.

Store in the back of the fridge

The back of the fridge is usually the coldest part, which is ideal for storing juice. Keeping the juice at a consistent low temperature will help slow down the growth of bacteria and prevent spoilage.

Fill the container completely

Fill the container completely with juice, leaving no air pockets. This will help prevent oxidation, which can cause the juice to lose its colour and flavour.

Label and date the container

Always label and date the container with the name of the juice and the date it was made. This will assist you in keeping track of how long it has been in the fridge and when it should be consumed.

Consume within 24-48 hours

Freshly made juice is best consumed within 24-48 hours of making it. After that, its nutritional value and flavour may start to decline. If you want to store your juice for longer periods, consider freezing it instead.

Avoid cross-contamination

Make sure to store your juice separately from other foods in the fridge to avoid cross-contamination. This will help prevent any bacteria from spreading to your juice and spoiling it.

Discard if signs of spoilage appear

If you notice any signs of spoilage, such as mould or an off smell, discard the juice immediately. Drinking spoiled juice can lead to foodborne illnesses, so it's better to be safe than sorry.

By following these simple guidelines, you can ensure that your freshly made juice stays fresh and safe to drink for longer periods in the fridge. Enjoy your healthy and delicious homemade juice!

Freezing your juice for later use

Freezing your juice is an excellent way to preserve its freshness and flavour for later use. Whether you're a health-conscious individual who likes to drink fresh juice daily or a busy parent who wants to provide their children with a healthy snack, freezing your juice can save you time and money.

Here are some advantages to freezing your juice:

1. Preserves Nutrients: When you freeze your juice, it locks in the nutrients and vitamins that would otherwise be lost during the oxidation process. This means that you'll be able to enjoy the same health benefits of your juice even after it's been frozen for several weeks.

2. Convenience: Freezing your juice allows you to have a healthy and refreshing drink on hand whenever you need it. You can simply take out a glassful from the freezer and let it thaw for a few minutes before drinking. This is especially convenient for busy individuals who don't have time to make fresh juice every day.

3. Cost-effective: Freezing your juice can help you save money in the long run. Instead of buying fresh juice every day, you can make a large batch of juice and freeze it in individual portions. This will not only save you money but also reduce food waste since you won't have to throw away any leftover juice.

4. Versatility: Frozen juice can be used in various ways, such as adding it to smoothies, using it as a base for popsicles, or blending it with other fruits to create a unique flavour profile. This versatility makes frozen juice an excellent ingredient for experimenting with new recipes and flavours.

Here are some tips for freezing your juice:

1. Use high-quality fruits: To ensure that your frozen juice tastes as good as fresh, use high-quality fruits that are ripe and in season. This will result in a more flavorful and nutritious juice that will freeze well.

2. Strain the juice: Before freezing your juice, strain out any pulp or sediment to prevent ice crystals from forming during the freezing process. This will also result in a smoother and more consistent texture when thawed.

3. Use an ice cube tray: Pour your strained juice into an ice cube tray and freeze until solid. This will allow you to easily thaw just the amount you need

without having to defrost the entire container of juice at once.

<u>4. Label and date the containers:</u> Once your frozen juice cubes are ready, transfer them to an airtight container or freezer bag and label them with the date of freezing. This will help you keep track of how long they've been in the freezer and ensure that they're consumed before they go bad.

In conclusion, freezing your juice is an excellent way to preserve its freshness, convenience, cost-effectiveness, and versatility for later use. By following these tips, you can enjoy delicious and healthy frozen juice that's just as good as fresh!

Preventing spoilage and mould growth

Spoilage and mould growth are common issues that can ruin the taste and quality of your freshly squeezed juice. Preventing these problems is crucial to preserve the juice's nutritional value and ensure its safety for consumption. Here are some tips to help you prevent spoilage and mould growth in your juice:

- Use fresh produce: The fresher the fruits and vegetables, the less likely they are to spoil or develop mould. Make sure to use produce that is ripe but not overripe, as this can lead to fermentation.

- Clean your equipment: Before squeezing your fruits and vegetables, clean your juicer thoroughly with hot water and soap. This will prevent any bacteria or mould spores from being transferred to the juice during the extraction process.

- Store your juice properly: After squeezing, store your juice in a clean, airtight container in the refrigerator. This will help prevent airborne bacteria from entering the container and causing spoilage. It's also important to consume the juice within 24-48 hours, as it can start to lose its nutritional value and flavor over time.

- Add lemon or lime juice: Adding a small amount of lemon or lime juice to your juice can help prevent spoilage by lowering the pH level, making it less hospitable for bacteria and mould.

- Freeze your juice: If you want to preserve your juice for longer than 24-48 hours, consider freezing it in ice cube trays or freezer bags. This will allow you to enjoy fresh juice at a later time without worrying about spoilage or mould growth.

- Use a straw: Using a straw can help prevent airborne bacteria from entering the container and contaminating the juice. This is especially important if you're sharing the juice with others or if you're using a communal glass or pitcher.

By following these tips, you can help prevent spoilage and mould growth in your homemade juice, ensuring that it stays fresh, delicious, and safe for consumption.

Recommended storage times for different types of juice

Proper storage is crucial to preserving the quality and freshness of juice. Different types of juice have varying storage times due to their natural acidity, sugar content, and potential for spoilage. Here are some recommended storage times for popular types of juice:

1. Orange Juice: Freshly squeezed orange juice should be consumed within 24 hours for optimal flavour and nutritional value. If stored in the refrigerator, it can last up to 5 days. However, the longer it sits, the more it will oxidise and lose its vibrant colour and flavour.

2. Apple Juice: Apple juice can be stored in the refrigerator for up to 2 weeks. It may develop a slightly sour taste over time due to its lower acidity compared to citrus juices. To prevent spoilage, make sure the juice is pasteurised before consumption.

3. Grape Juice: Grape juice can last up to 3 weeks in the refrigerator if unopened. Once opened, it should be consumed within 1 week to prevent mould growth. Grape juice is naturally sweeter than orange or apple juice, which can lead to faster spoilage if not stored properly.

4. Pineapple Juice: Pineapple juice should be consumed within 5 days of opening due to its high sugar content and susceptibility to spoilage. If you want to extend its shelf life, freeze it in ice cube trays and use it in smoothies or cocktails later on.

5. Cranberry Juice: Cranberry juice can last up to 2 weeks in the refrigerator if unopened. Once opened, it should be consumed within 1 week due to its low acidity and potential for spoilage. Cranberry juice may also separate over time due to its high fibre content, so give it a good shake before drinking.

6. Carrot Juice: Carrot juice can last up to 5 days in the refrigerator due to its high vitamin C content and natural preservatives. However, it may develop a slightly bitter taste over time due to oxidation. To prevent this, store it in a dark container and consume it as soon as possible after opening.

7. Beet Juice: Beet juice can last up to 3 days in the refrigerator due to its high sugar content and potential for spoilage. It may also stain your refrigerator shelves or containers, so consider using glass bottles with tight-fitting lids or opaque containers to prevent discoloration.

In general, it's best to consume freshly squeezed juice as soon as possible for optimal flavour and nutrition. If you prefer longer shelf life, consider freezing your juice in ice cube trays or purchasing pasteurised juices from the store for added safety and convenience.

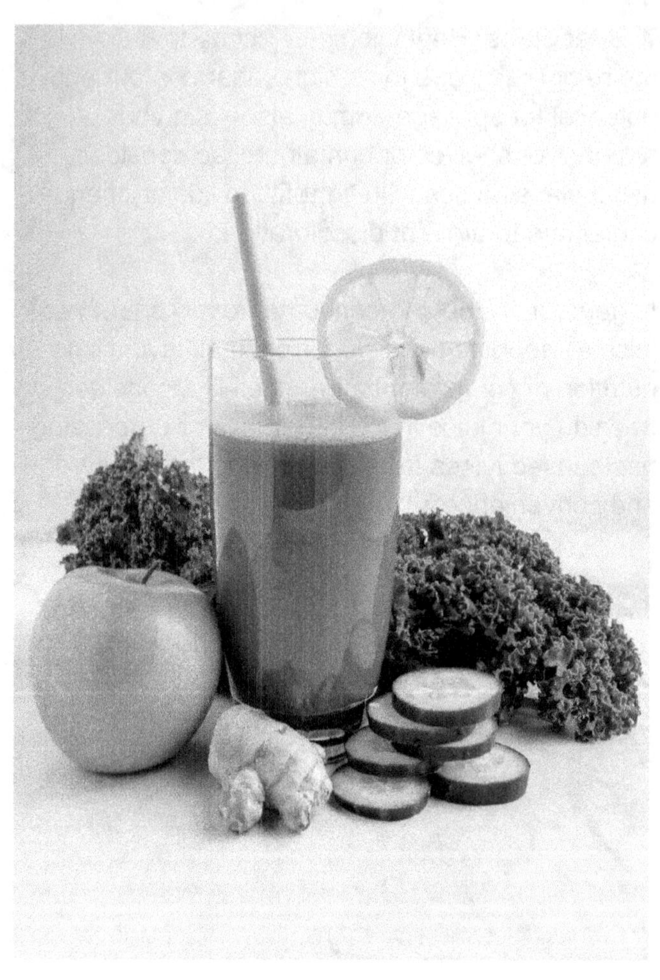

CHAPTER FOUR

Juicing Tips and Tricks

How to adjust the consistency of your juice to suit your preferences

Adjusting the consistency of your juice to suit your preferences is a simple process that can make a big difference in the overall taste and texture of your drink. Here are some tips on how to achieve the consistency you desire:

- Start with the right ingredients: The type of fruits and vegetables you choose will have a significant impact on the consistency of your juice. For a thicker juice, use more fibrous ingredients like apples, carrots, and beets. For a thinner juice, use more watery ingredients like cucumber, celery, and lettuce.

- Adjust the amount of liquid: The amount of liquid you add to your juicer will also affect the consistency of your juice. Use less liquid for a thicker juice, and more liquid for a thinner juice. You can also use water as a base instead of fruit or vegetable juice to

make your juice less sweet and more
watery.

- Experiment with different ratios: Try mixing
  different fruits and vegetables in varying
  ratios to find the perfect consistency for your
  taste buds. For example, you could try using
  two apples and one beet for a thicker juice,
  or four cucumbers and two celery stalks for
  a thinner juice.

- Use a blender: If you prefer a thicker, pulpy
  juice, consider using a blender instead of a
  juicer. Blending will break down the fibres in
  the fruits and vegetables, creating a thicker,
  creamier texture. You can also add ice or
  frozen fruit to create a slushie-like
  consistency.

- Strain the pulp: If you prefer a smoother,
  less pulpy juice, strain out the solids using a
  fine-mesh strainer or cheesecloth. This will
  remove any remaining fibres and create a
  smoother texture.

- Adjust the sweetness: The sweetness level
  of your juice can also affect its consistency.
  Use sweeter fruits like apples or pineapples
  to create a thicker, more syrupy juice, or use
  less sweet fruits like cucumber or celery for
  a thinner, more refreshing juice.

Remember that everyone's preferences are different, so it may take some experimentation to find the perfect consistency for you. Don't be afraid to try new combinations and ratios until you find what works best for your taste buds!

How to add variety to your juice routine with different fruits and vegetables

Adding variety to your juice routine with different fruits and vegetables can not only make your daily intake more exciting but also provide your body with a wider range of essential nutrients. Here are some tips on how to add variety to your juice routine:

1. Experiment with different fruits and vegetables: Don't be afraid to try new things! Some great options for adding variety to your juices include kale, spinach, cucumber, beetroot, carrot, apple, orange, lemon, ginger, and turmeric. You can also mix and match different fruits and vegetables to create unique flavour combinations.

2. Use seasonal produce: Seasonal fruits and vegetables are often fresher and more flavorful than those that are out of season. Plus, they're typically less expensive. Check out what's in season in your area and incorporate those items into your juice routine.

3. Add superfoods: Superfoods like acai berries, goji berries, chia seeds, and spirulina can add a nutritional boost to your juices. Just be sure to use them in moderation as they can be high in calories and fibre.

4. Use herbs and spices: Herbs like mint, basil, and cilantro can add a fresh burst of flavour to your juices. Spices like cinnamon, nutmeg, and cumin can add warmth and depth of flavour. Just be sure to use them sparingly as they can be overpowering in large quantities.

5. Don't forget about hydration: Juicing is a great way to get hydrated, but it's also important to drink plenty of water throughout the day. Try adding lemon or cucumber slices to your water for an extra burst of flavour.

6. Keep it balanced: When creating your juice recipes, aim for a balance of carbohydrates, protein, and fat. This will keep you full and satisfied in between meals. Some great options for adding protein include almond butter or chia seeds, while avocado is a great source of healthy fats.

7. Store excess juice: If you find yourself with more juice than you can drink at once, store it in the refrigerator for up to 24 hours. This will allow you to enjoy the benefits of the juice over a longer period of time.

By following these tips, you'll be able to add variety to your juice routine while still reaping the many health benefits that come with drinking fresh fruit and vegetable juices!

Tips for storing your juice to ensure maximum nutritional value and freshness

Juicing is a popular trend in the health and wellness industry due to its numerous health benefits. However, to ensure maximum nutritional value and freshness, it's essential to store your juice correctly. Here are some storage suggestions for your juice:

1. Store your juice in airtight containers:

To prevent oxidation, which can cause your juice to lose its nutritional value and flavour, store your juice in airtight containers. This will also prevent any contamination from airborne bacteria.

2. Keep your juice cold:

Cold temperatures help preserve the nutrients in your juice, as well as prevent bacterial growth. Store your juice in the refrigerator immediately after juicing, and consume it within 24-48 hours.

3. Use glass containers:

Glass containers are a better option than plastic or metal containers because they don't leach chemicals into the juice, which can affect its taste and nutritional value. Glass containers are also easy to clean and reuse.

4. Avoid storing your juice for too long:

While it's possible to store your juice for up to 72 hours, it's best to consume it as soon as possible after juicing to ensure maximum nutritional value and freshness. The more nutrients that are lost as the juice sits, the longer it sits.

5. Shake before consuming:

As the juice separates over time, shake it before consuming to ensure that all the ingredients are well mixed. This will also help distribute any sediment that may have settled at the bottom of the container.

6. Use high-quality produce:

The quality of the produce you use affects the nutritional value and freshness of your juice. Always use fresh, organic produce whenever possible to ensure maximum nutritional value and freshness.

7. Clean your juicer thoroughly:

After juicing, clean your juicer thoroughly with hot water and soap to prevent any bacteria buildup that could affect the quality of your next batch of juice. This will also help prevent any off flavours or odours from carrying over into future batches of juice.

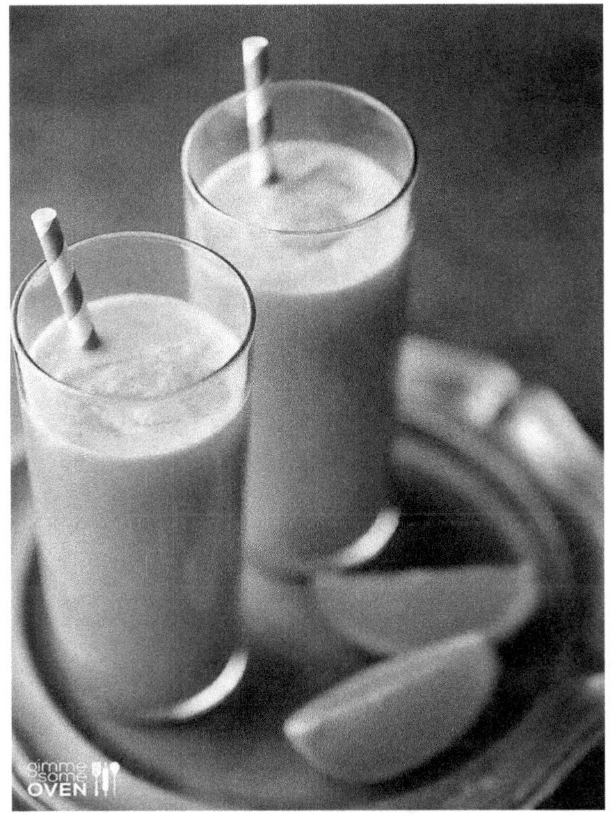

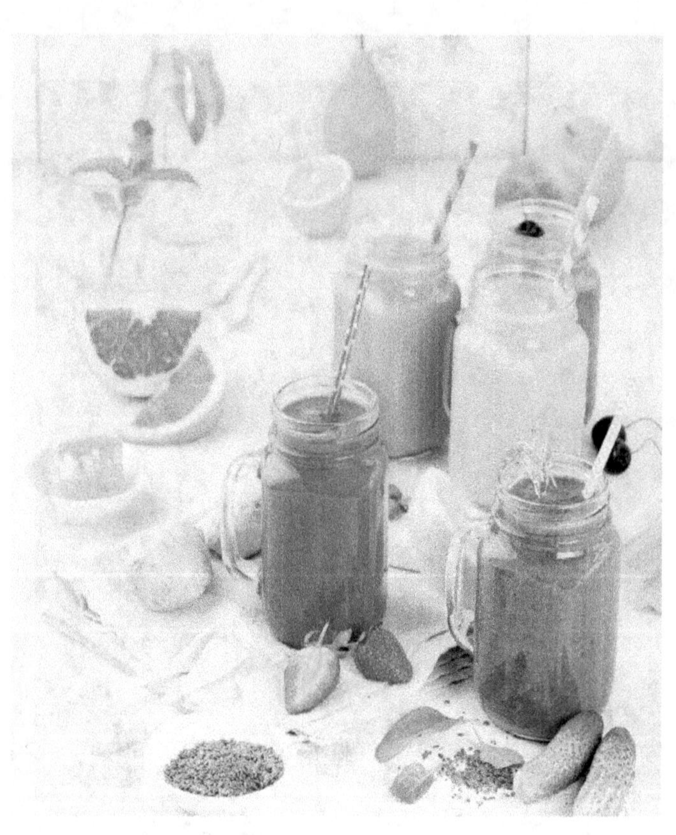

CHAPTER FIVE

Juicing Benefits and Risks

The potential health benefits of juicing, such as increased nutrient absorption and improved digestion

Juicing has gained immense popularity in recent years as a health trend, and for good reason. Juicing involves extracting the liquid content of fruits and vegetables and discarding the pulp, resulting in a nutrient-dense beverage that is packed with vitamins, minerals, and antioxidants. Here are some potential health benefits of juicing:

1. Increased Nutrient Absorption:

When we eat whole fruits and vegetables, our bodies have to work hard to break down the fibre and extract the nutrients. This can sometimes result in less than optimal absorption of nutrients. However, when we juice, the fibre is removed, making it easier for our bodies to absorb the nutrients. This is particularly beneficial for individuals with digestive issues or those who have difficulty consuming large amounts of fibre.

2. Improved Digestion:

While fibre is important for overall digestive health, some individuals may experience discomfort or bloating due to high fibre intake. Juicing allows us to consume a large amount of fruits and vegetables without the added fibre, making it easier on the digestive system. Additionally, certain fruits and vegetables that are difficult to digest when eaten whole, such as beets and carrots, are easier to digest when juiced.

3. Increased Hydration:

Many fruits and vegetables are high in water content, making them an excellent source of hydration. When we juice these foods, we are able to consume a large amount of water along with the nutrients, which can help to prevent dehydration and promote overall health.

4. Increased Energy:

Juicing can provide a quick burst of energy due to the high concentration of nutrients in a small volume. This can be particularly beneficial for individuals who lead busy lifestyles or have limited time for meal preparation. Additionally, because juices are easily digested, they can provide an immediate source of energy without causing a spike in blood sugar levels.

Many fruits and vegetables are rich in antioxidants, which can help to protect our skin from damage caused by free radicals. When we juice these foods, we are able to consume a large amount of antioxidants in a single serving, which can help to improve overall skin health and prevent signs of ageing.

In conclusion, juicing offers numerous potential health benefits due to its high concentration of nutrients and ease of digestion. Whether you are looking to improve your overall health or address specific health concerns, incorporating juicing into your diet may be a beneficial addition to your lifestyle. As with any dietary change, it is always recommended to consult with a healthcare professional before making significant changes to your diet.

The risks associated with juicing, such as high sugar content in some fruits and vegetable combinations

Juicing has gained immense popularity in recent years as a healthy and convenient way to consume fruits and vegetables. While juicing can provide numerous health benefits, it's essential to be aware of the potential risks associated with this practice. One of the most significant risks is the high sugar content in some fruit and vegetable combinations.

Fruits are naturally sweet, and when they're juiced, the fibre that helps regulate blood sugar levels is removed. This can lead to a rapid spike in blood sugar levels, which can result in energy crashes and cravings for sugary foods. Moreover, consuming too many high-sugar fruits in one sitting can contribute to weight gain, obesity, and other related health issues.

For instance, carrot-orange juice is a popular combination that's high in sugar due to the high sugar content in oranges. Similarly, beetroot-apple juice is also high in sugar due to the sweetness of apples. While these fruits are healthy when consumed in moderation, it's essential to balance them with low-sugar vegetables like kale, spinach, and cucumber to prevent a sugar overload.

Another risk associated with juicing is the potential for nutrient loss during the juicing process. When fruits and vegetables are juiced, they're stripped of their fibre content, which can lead to the loss of essential nutrients like vitamins A, C, and E. This is because fibre helps the body absorb these vitamins more efficiently. Therefore, it's crucial to consume whole fruits and vegetables instead of relying solely on juice for nutrition.

Moreover, some people may experience digestive issues when consuming large amounts of juice due to its high acidity level. This can lead to indigestion, bloating, and acid reflux. To prevent these issues, it's recommended to drink juice slowly and in moderation.

In conclusion, while juicing can provide numerous health benefits when done correctly, it's essential to be aware of the potential risks associated with this practice. Consuming high-sugar fruit combinations can lead to energy crashes and weight gain, while nutrient loss during the juicing process can result in a lack of essential nutrients. To mitigate these risks, it's recommended to balance high-sugar fruits with low-sugar vegetables and consume whole fruits and vegetables instead of relying solely on juice for nutrition. Additionally, it's crucial to drink juice slowly and in moderation to prevent digestive issues. By following these guidelines, individuals can enjoy the benefits of juicing while minimising its risks.

How to balance the benefits and risks of juicing to achieve optimal health outcomes

Juicing has gained immense popularity in recent years as a way to promote optimal health outcomes. While there are numerous benefits to juicing, such as increased nutrient intake, improved digestion, and enhanced energy levels, it's essential to balance the benefits with the potential risks. Here are some tips on how to achieve optimal health outcomes through juicing while minimising the risks:

Choose the right fruits and vegetables:

Not all fruits and vegetables are created equal. Some are high in sugar, while others are low in fibre. It's crucial to select fruits and vegetables that are rich in nutrients and low in sugar. Some excellent options include kale, spinach, cucumber, celery, apples, carrots, and ginger.

Balance sweetness with bitterness:

While sweet fruits like apples and oranges can make your juice taste delicious, they're also high in sugar. To balance the sweetness, add bitter vegetables like kale or celery to your juice. This will not only improve the flavour but also help regulate blood sugar levels.

Don't overdo it:

While juicing can be a great way to pack in a lot of nutrients at once, it's essential not to overdo it. Consuming too many fruits and vegetables in juice form can lead to an overload of fibre and sugar, which can cause digestive issues like bloating and diarrhoea. Stick to one or two servings of juice per day and consume the rest of your fruits and vegetables whole.

Use a high-quality juicer:

Investing in a high-quality juicer is crucial for achieving optimal health outcomes through juicing. A good juicer will extract as many nutrients as possible from your fruits and vegetables while minimising waste. Look for a juicer that uses a slow speed extraction process to preserve the enzymes and nutrients in your produce.

Store your juice properly:

Juice should be consumed within 24 hours of preparation to ensure maximum nutrient content. Store your juice in an airtight container in the refrigerator and consume it as soon as possible. If you must store it for longer than 24 hours, freeze it in ice cube trays and use it as needed.

Consult with a healthcare professional:

If you have any underlying health conditions or are taking medications that could interact with certain fruits and vegetables, it's essential to consult with a healthcare professional before starting a juicing regimen. They can provide guidance on which fruits and vegetables are safe for you to consume and how often you should be juicing.

By following these tips, you can balance the benefits and risks of juicing to achieve optimal health outcomes while minimising the potential risks. Remember to always listen to your body and make adjustments as needed based on how you feel after consuming your juice.

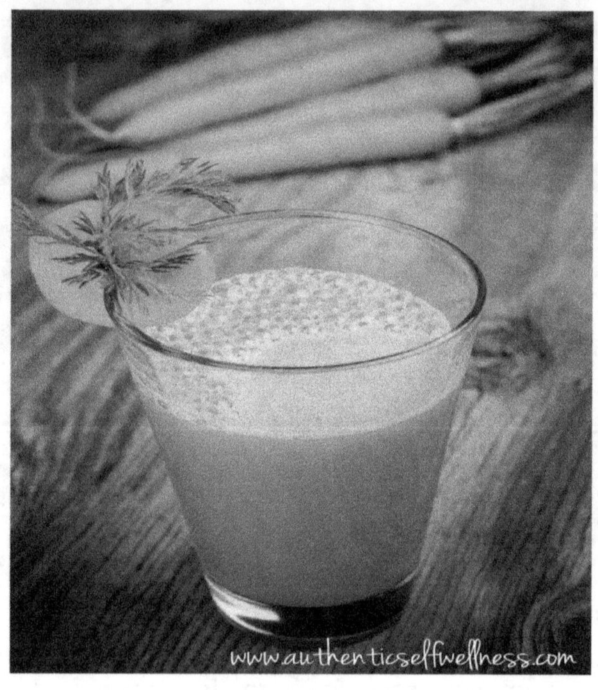

CHAPTER SIX

Health Benefits of Juicing and How to Maximise Them

Boosting your immune system with vitamins and minerals

Juicing has gained immense popularity in recent years as a healthy and convenient way to consume an array of vitamins and minerals that can boost the immune system. Juicing involves extracting the liquid content of fruits and vegetables, leaving behind the fibre. This process makes it easier for the body to absorb the nutrients, as they are in a more bioavailable form. In this article, we will explore some of the key vitamins and minerals found in juices that can enhance immunity and how they contribute to overall health benefits.

Vitamin C:

Vitamin C is a powerful antioxidant that plays a crucial role in boosting immunity. It helps to protect the body from free radicals, which can damage cells and contribute to chronic diseases such as cancer and heart disease. Citrus fruits including oranges, lemons, limes, and grapefruits are high in vitamin C. Other fruits rich in vitamin C include strawberries, kiwis, papayas, and bell peppers.

Vitamin A:

Vitamin A is essential for maintaining a healthy immune system. It helps to promote the growth and development of white blood cells, which are responsible for fighting off infections. Foods rich in vitamin A include carrots, sweet potatoes, spinach, kale, and mangoes.

Vitamin E:

Vitamin E is another antioxidant that helps to protect the body from damage caused by free radicals. It also plays a role in supporting the immune system by promoting the production of white blood cells. Foods rich in vitamin E include avocados, almonds, sunflower seeds, and spinach.

Minerals:

In addition to vitamins, juices also contain a variety of minerals that contribute to overall health benefits. Here are a few of the most important:

Potassium:

Potassium is an essential mineral that aids in blood pressure regulation and heart function. It also plays a role in maintaining proper muscle function.

Bananas, sweet potatoes, spinach, and avocados are high in potassium.

Magnesium:

Magnesium is involved in over 300 biochemical reactions in the body and is essential for maintaining proper nerve and muscle function. It also helps to maintain bone health. Foods rich in magnesium include leafy greens such as spinach and kale, almonds, avocados, and bananas.

Iron:

Iron is essential for maintaining proper red blood cell function and preventing anaemia. Foods rich in iron include leafy greens such as spinach and kale, beets, apples, and carrots. Vitamin C-rich foods such as citrus fruits can also help to enhance iron absorption.

Maximising Immune System Benefits:

To maximise the immune system benefits of juicing, it's essential to choose a variety of fruits and vegetables that are rich in vitamins and minerals. Here are some tips for creating immune-boosting juices:

1) Choose a variety of colourful fruits and vegetables to ensure you're getting a range of vitamins and minerals.

 2) Include citrus fruits such as oranges or lemons to enhance iron absorption from leafy greens like spinach or kale.

3) Add ginger or turmeric for their anti-inflammatory properties.

4) Use organic produce whenever possible to avoid exposure to pesticides and other chemicals that can weaken the immune system.

5) Drink your juice immediately after making it to ensure maximum nutrient absorption.

In conclusion, juicing is an excellent way to consume a variety of vitamins and minerals that can boost immunity and support overall health benefits.
By choosing a variety of colourful fruits and vegetables and maximising nutrient absorption through techniques like adding citrus fruits or using organic produce, you can create delicious immune-boosting juices that will leave you feeling healthy and energised!

Improving digestion and nutrient absorption

Juicing has gained immense popularity in recent years as a healthy and convenient way to consume a variety of fruits and vegetables.
Not only does juicing provide a quick and easy source of nutrients, but it also offers several health benefits, including improving digestion and enhancing nutrient absorption.

Digestion is the process by which our bodies break down food into nutrients that can be absorbed and utilised.
A healthy digestive system is essential for maintaining overall health and preventing diseases. Juicing can significantly improve digestion in several ways:

1. Increases fibre intake: Although juices do not contain the fibre-rich pulp found in whole fruits and vegetables, they still provide a significant amount of fibre. Fibre is essential for maintaining a healthy digestive system as it helps to prevent constipation, regulate bowel movements, and reduce the risk of colon cancer.

2. Promotes hydration: Juices are rich in water content, making them an excellent source of hydration. Dehydration can lead to constipation, which can negatively impact digestion. By consuming enough water through juicing, we can ensure that our bodies remain hydrated, promoting healthy digestion.

3. Reduces bloating: Many people experience bloating after consuming certain foods, which can negatively impact digestion. Juicing allows us to remove the high-fibre content found in whole fruits and vegetables, making it easier for our bodies to digest the nutrients without causing bloating or discomfort.

4. Reduces inflammation: Many chronic diseases, such as inflammatory bowel disease (IBD), are associated with inflammation in the gut. Juicing provides anti-inflammatory nutrients such as vitamin C, beta-carotene, and omega-3 fatty acids that can help reduce inflammation in the gut, promoting healthy digestion.

In addition to improving digestion, juicing also enhances nutrient absorption by providing a concentrated source of vitamins, minerals, and other essential nutrients. When we consume whole fruits and vegetables, our bodies must expend energy to break down the fibrous cell walls and extract the nutrients. By juicing, we remove these cell walls, making it easier for our bodies to absorb the nutrients directly into the bloodstream.
This process is known as "juice therapy" or "juice cleansing" and has been shown to have several health benefits:

☐ Increases nutrient intake: Juicing allows us to consume a higher concentration of vitamins, minerals, and other essential nutrients than we would through whole fruits and vegetables alone. This increased intake can help prevent deficiencies and promote overall health.

☐ Improves nutrient bioavailability: By removing the fibre from whole fruits and vegetables during juicing, we increase the bioavailability of certain nutrients such as iron, calcium, and vitamin C. This increased bioavailability allows our bodies to absorb these nutrients more efficiently than they would through whole foods alone.

☐ Enhances detoxification: Many people use juicing as a way to detoxify their bodies by consuming large amounts of fruits and vegetables rich in antioxidants and other detoxifying compounds such as chlorophyll and glucosinolates. These compounds help to eliminate toxins from the body, promoting overall health and wellbeing.

In conclusion, juicing offers several health benefits, including improving digestion and enhancing nutrient absorption. By increasing fibre intake, promoting hydration, reducing bloating, and reducing inflammation through juicing, we can improve our digestive health significantly. Additionally, by increasing nutrient intake, improving nutrient bioavailability, and enhancing detoxification through juice therapy or juice cleansing, we can promote overall health and wellbeing. It's essential to remember that while juicing offers many benefits, it should be consumed in moderation as part of a balanced diet to ensure that we are meeting all of our nutritional needs.

Reducing inflammation and oxidative stress

Juicing has gained immense popularity in recent years as a health trend due to its numerous benefits. One of the most significant advantages of juicing is its ability to reduce inflammation and oxidative stress in the body. Inflammation and oxidative stress are two major factors that contribute to various chronic diseases such as cancer, heart disease, and Alzheimer's. In this article, we will discuss how juicing can help reduce inflammation and oxidative stress and how to maximise these health benefits.

The body's natural response to injury or infection is inflammation. Chronic inflammation, on the other hand, can cause tissue damage and contribute to the development of illnesses. Oxidative stress, on the other hand, occurs when there is an imbalance between the production of free radicals and the body's ability to detoxify them. Free radicals are unstable chemicals that can harm cells and accelerate the ageing and disease process.

Juicing can help reduce inflammation and oxidative stress in several ways:

- Antioxidant-rich fruits and vegetables: Many fruits and vegetables contain antioxidants that can help neutralise free radicals and reduce oxidative stress. Some examples of antioxidant-rich fruits and vegetables that are great for juicing include berries, kale, spinach, beets, carrots, and ginger.

- Anti-inflammatory compounds: Some fruits and vegetables also contain anti-inflammatory compounds that can help reduce inflammation in the body. Turmeric, for example, contains a compound called curcumin that has been shown to have anti-inflammatory properties. Other anti-inflammatory fruits and vegetables include pineapple, papaya, cucumber, celery, and parsley.

- Enzymes: Juicing also helps preserve the enzymes found in fruits and vegetables, which can aid in digestion and reduce inflammation. Enzymes such as bromelain (found in pineapple) and papain (found in papaya) have been shown to have anti-inflammatory properties.

To maximise the health benefits of juicing for reducing inflammation and oxidative stress, here are some tips:

1. Choose a variety of fruits and vegetables: Incorporate a mix of antioxidant-rich fruits and vegetables as well as anti-inflammatory compounds into your juice recipes. This will ensure that you are getting a wide range of nutrients that can help reduce inflammation and oxidative stress.

2. Use organic produce: Organic produce is less likely to contain pesticides or other chemicals that can contribute to inflammation and oxidative stress. If organic produce is not available or affordable, consider washing your produce thoroughly before juicing.

3. Add ginger: Ginger has anti-inflammatory properties and can also help improve digestion. Adding a small piece of ginger to your juice recipe can help enhance its health benefits.

4. Drink your juice immediately: Juice is best consumed immediately after preparation to ensure that it retains its nutrients and enzymes. If you cannot drink your juice right away, store it in an airtight container in the refrigerator for up to 24 hours.

5. Consult with a healthcare professional: If you have a chronic disease or are taking medication for an existing condition, it is always best to consult with a healthcare professional before making significant changes to your diet or lifestyle habits. They can provide personalised advice based on your individual needs and circumstances.

Promoting healthy weight loss and detoxification

For good reason, juicing has become a hot fad in the health and wellness business. Not only does it provide a convenient and delicious way to consume fruits and vegetables, but it also offers numerous health benefits, including promoting healthy weight loss and detoxification.

Healthy Weight Loss

One of the most significant benefits of juicing for weight loss is that it helps to reduce calorie intake. Fruits and vegetables are low in calories but high in fibre, vitamins, and minerals, making them an ideal choice for weight loss. By consuming a variety of fruits and vegetables in their liquid form, individuals can consume a high volume of nutrients without consuming too many calories.

Moreover, juicing can help to curb cravings for unhealthy foods. When we consume processed or high-calorie foods, our bodies release dopamine, a feel-good hormone that can lead to cravings. By consuming nutrient-dense foods like fruits and vegetables, we can satisfy our cravings for sweet or savoury flavours without consuming excess calories.

Detoxification

Another significant benefit of juicing is its ability to aid in detoxification. Our bodies naturally detoxify themselves through the liver, kidneys, and digestive system. However, our modern diets often contain processed foods, chemicals, and toxins that can overburden these organs. Juicing can help to support the body's natural detoxification process by providing it with the nutrients it needs to eliminate toxins efficiently.

Fruits and vegetables contain antioxidants, which help to neutralise free radicals in the body that can cause oxidative stress and damage cells. Leafy greens like spinach and kale are rich in chlorophyll, which helps to purify the blood and support liver function. Ginger and lemon are also excellent additions to a juice as they aid in digestion and stimulate the production of bile, which helps to eliminate toxins from the body.

To maximise the health benefits of juicing for weight loss and detoxification, there are a few tips to follow:

1. Choose a variety of fruits and vegetables: Consuming a variety of colours ensures that you are getting a wide range of vitamins, minerals, and antioxidants.

2. Include leafy greens: Leafy greens like spinach, kale, and collard greens are low in calories but high in fibre, vitamins, and minerals. They also contain chlorophyll, which helps to purify the blood and support liver function.

3. Add ginger and lemon: Ginger has anti-inflammatory properties that help to reduce bloating and aid in digestion. Lemon is rich in vitamin C and helps to stimulate the production of bile, which helps to eliminate toxins from the body.

4. Drink your juice slowly: Sipping your juice slowly allows your body time to absorb the nutrients fully. It also helps you feel more satisfied as you consume your juice over a longer period.

5. Consume your juice as part of a healthy diet: While juicing can be an excellent addition to a healthy diet, it should not replace whole foods entirely. Consuming whole fruits and vegetables provides additional fibre that is essential for maintaining a healthy weight and promoting overall health.

Juicing tips for incorporating it into a healthy lifestyle

Juicing has grown in popularity as a means to include more fruits and vegetables into our diets in recent years.
Not only does juicing provide a quick and convenient way to consume nutrients, but it can also help improve overall health and wellbeing. Here are some tips for incorporating juicing into a healthy lifestyle:

1. Start slow: If you're new to juicing, it's essential to start slow and gradually increase your intake. Begin with one or two servings per day and work your way up as your body adjusts to the new routine.

2. Choose the right ingredients: When selecting fruits and vegetables for juicing, opt for those that are high in nutrients and low in sugar. Some excellent options include kale, spinach, cucumber, celery, carrots, ginger, and lemon.

3. Balance your juices: To ensure a balanced diet, aim to include a variety of fruits and vegetables in your juices. This will provide a range of vitamins, minerals, and fibre that your body needs.

4. Don't forget the greens: Leafy greens like kale, spinach, and collard greens are packed with nutrients like vitamin C, vitamin K, and iron. Incorporate them into your juices to reap their benefits.

5. Add some spice: Ginger and turmeric are both anti-inflammatory spices that can add flavour and health benefits to your juices. Try adding a small piece of fresh ginger or a pinch of turmeric to your next juice for an extra boost.

6. Use a high-quality juicer: Investing in a high-quality juicer can make all the difference in the quality of your juices. Look for one that extracts as much juice as possible while preserving the nutrients and fibre.

7. Store your juice properly: If you're not going to drink your juice right away, store it in an airtight container in the refrigerator for up to 24 hours. This will help prevent spoilage and ensure that the nutrients remain intact.

8. Don't replace meals with juice: While juicing can be a healthy addition to your diet, it should not replace meals entirely. Stick to using it as a supplement to your regular meals to ensure that you're getting all the nutrients your body needs.

9. Stay hydrated: Juicing can be dehydrating due to the lack of fibre in the fruits and vegetables used. Make sure to drink plenty of water throughout the day to stay hydrated and prevent dehydration-related issues like headaches and dizziness.

10. Enjoy the process: Juicing should be an enjoyable experience that you look forward to each day. Experiment with different combinations of fruits and vegetables to find what works best for you, and don't be afraid to get creative!

Common Misconceptions about Juicing

Juicing has gained immense popularity in recent years as a health trend, with many people turning to this method of consuming fruits and vegetables as a way to boost their nutrient intake and improve their overall well-being. However, there are several common misconceptions about juicing that need to be addressed.

- Juicing is a quick fix for weight loss: While juicing can be a helpful tool for weight loss, it is not a magic solution. Juices are low in fibre, which means that they can cause blood sugar spikes and crashes, leading to hunger and overeating. Additionally, juices are often high in calories due to the large volume of fruits used, making it easy to

consume too many calories. A healthy
weight loss plan should include a balanced
diet, regular exercise, and lifestyle changes.

- Juicing is a substitute for whole fruits and
  vegetables: While juicing can be a
  convenient way to consume large amounts
  of fruits and vegetables at once, it is not a
  substitute for whole foods. Whole fruits and
  vegetables contain fibre, which is essential
  for digestion and helps to keep you feeling
  full. Fibre also slows down the absorption of
  sugar into the bloodstream, preventing
  spikes in blood sugar levels. By consuming
  whole fruits and vegetables instead of
  juices, you can also enjoy the texture and
  chewing experience that comes with eating
  whole foods.

- Juicing is expensive: While it is true that
  some high-end juicers can be expensive,
  there are many affordable options available
  on the market. Additionally, you can save
  money by buying fruits and vegetables in
  bulk or growing your own produce. Juicing
  also allows you to use parts of the fruit or
  vegetable that might otherwise go to waste,
  such as the stems or leaves. By being
  creative with your ingredients and using
  what you have on hand, you can make
  delicious and nutritious juices without
  breaking the bank.

- Juicing is unhealthy because it removes fibre: While it is true that juicing removes the fibre from fruits and vegetables, this does not necessarily make it unhealthy. Fibre is important for digestion and preventing constipation, but it is not essential for nutrient absorption. In fact, some people with digestive issues find that removing the fibre from their fruits and vegetables makes it easier to digest and absorb the nutrients more efficiently. Additionally, you can add fibre back into your juice by blending in some leafy greens or adding chia seeds or flax seeds as a thickener.

- Juicing requires a lot of time: While it is true that preparing fresh juices can take some time, there are many ways to make the process more efficient. You can batch prepare your juices at the beginning of the week and store them in the fridge for later consumption. You can also invest in a slow juicer or a centrifugal juicer with a large capacity tank to reduce the amount of time spent cleaning up after each juice session. By being organised and efficient with your juicing routine, you can save time while still enjoying all the benefits of freshly made juices.

In conclusion, while juicing has its benefits, it is important to approach it with a balanced perspective. Juicing should be seen as a complementary part of a healthy lifestyle rather than a substitute for whole foods or a quick fix for weight loss or other health issues. By being mindful of portion sizes, incorporating whole foods into your diet, and being creative with your ingredients, you can enjoy all the benefits of freshly made juices without falling prey to common misconceptions about this popular health trend.

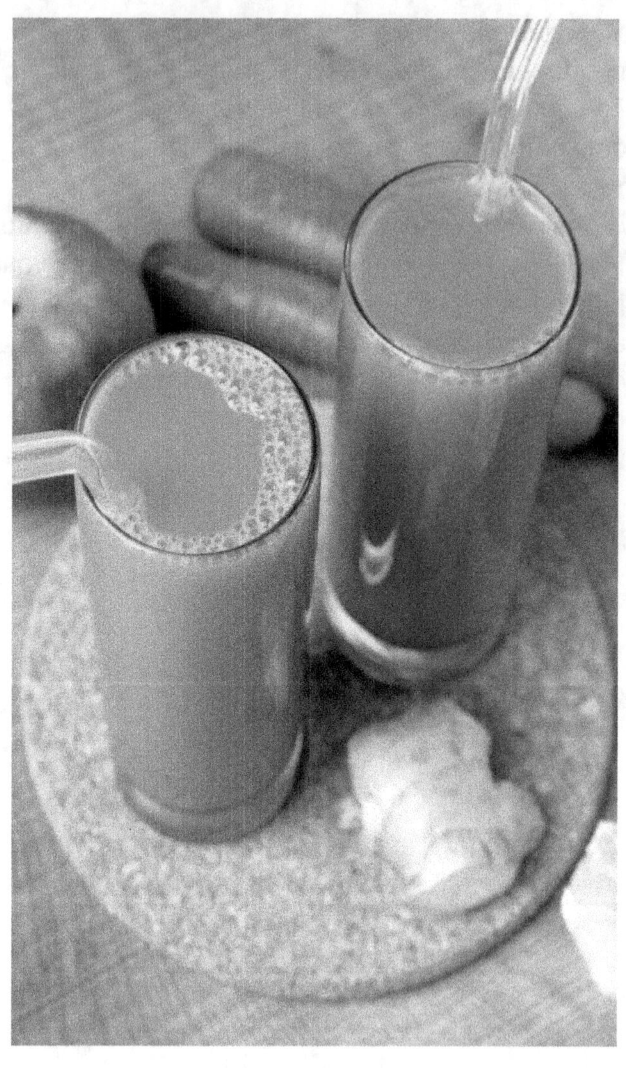

CONCLUSION

Summary of key takeaways from this guide on juicing for beginners

This guide on juicing for beginners provides several key takeaways that can help individuals embark on their juicing journey. Here are a few of the most significant:

Understand the benefits of juicing:

Juicing allows your body to absorb nutrients more easily and quickly than eating whole fruits and vegetables. It can also help you consume more fruits and vegetables in a single serving, which is essential for maintaining a healthy diet.

Choose the right equipment:

Invest in a high-quality juicer that can handle a variety of fruits and vegetables. Look for one with adjustable settings to customise your juice's texture and consistency.

Start with simple recipes:

Begin by juicing basic fruits and vegetables such as apples, carrots, and spinach. Gradually add more complex ingredients as you become more comfortable with the process.

Clean your equipment properly:

After each use, thoroughly clean your juicer to prevent bacteria buildup and ensure longevity.

Store your juice properly:

Store your juice in an airtight container in the refrigerator for up to 24 hours. Avoid storing it for too long, as it can lose its nutritional value over time.

Experiment with different flavours:

Don't be afraid to mix and match different fruits and vegetables to create unique and delicious juice blends.

Listen to your body:

Pay attention to how your body reacts to different juice combinations. Some people may experience digestive issues or sugar crashes from certain ingredients, so it's essential to find what works best for you.

Make juicing a part of your daily routine:

Incorporate juicing into your daily routine by setting aside time each day to prepare your juice. This will help you develop a consistent habit and reap the full benefits of juicing.

Encouragement to continue exploring the world of juicing as a way to promote a healthy lifestyle.

As we navigate through the hustle and bustle of daily life, it's easy to forget about the importance of taking care of our bodies. With the rise of fast-food culture and sedentary lifestyles, it's no surprise that many of us are struggling with our health. However, there is a simple and delicious way to promote a healthy lifestyle - juicing.

Juicing involves extracting the liquid content from fruits and vegetables, leaving behind the fibre. This process allows your body to absorb the nutrients more easily and quickly, making it an excellent addition to your daily routine. If you're new to juicing or have been hesitant to give it a try, here are a few reasons why you should continue exploring this world:

1. Packed with Nutrients:

Fruits and vegetables are loaded with essential vitamins, minerals, and antioxidants that our bodies need to function properly. Juicing allows you to consume a large amount of these nutrients in one glass, making it an easy way to meet your daily requirements.

2. Boosts Energy:

Because juices are easily digestible, they provide a quick energy boost without the crash that comes with consuming sugary drinks or processed foods. This makes them an excellent option for those who need a pick-me-up during the day.

3. Promotes Weight Loss:

Juices are low in calories and high in fibre, making them an excellent choice for those looking to shed a few pounds. By replacing sugary drinks and processed snacks with fresh juices, you can significantly reduce your calorie intake while still feeling satisfied.

4. Improves Digestion:

The fibre in fruits and vegetables is essential for maintaining a healthy digestive system. By consuming fresh juices regularly, you can help keep your digestive system running smoothly and prevent issues like constipation and bloating.

5. Encourages Creativity:

Juicing allows you to get creative in the kitchen by combining different fruits and vegetables in unique ways. This can be a fun and exciting way to experiment with new flavours and find what works best for your body.

In conclusion, there are countless benefits to incorporating juicing into your daily routine. From boosting energy to promoting weight loss and improving digestion, there's no denying that this trend is here to stay. So why not give it a try? Whether you're new to juicing or a seasoned pro, there's always something new to discover in this exciting world of health and wellness. Cheers to a happy and healthy lifestyle!

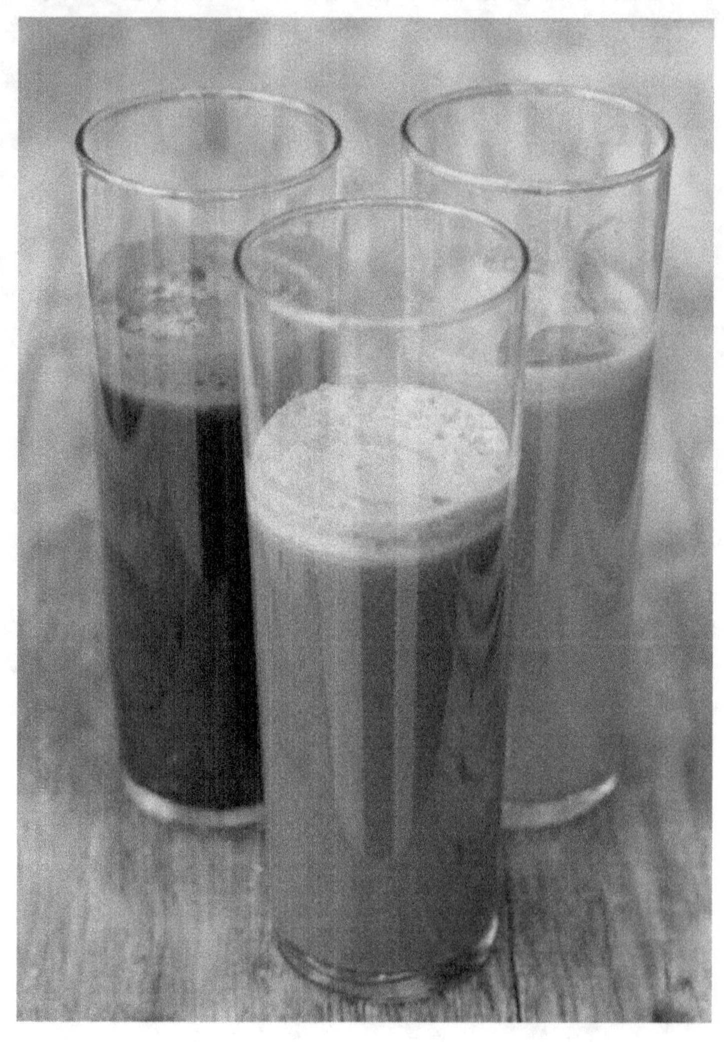